Entrancing Tales for Change with Hypnosis and NLP

by

The English Sisters

Violeta Zuggo, Jutka Zuggo

First edition published in 2011
© Copyright 2011
Violeta Zuggo, Jutka Zuggo

The right of Violeta Zuggo and Jutka Zuggo to be identified as the author of this work has been asserted by them in accordance with the Copyright, Designs and Patents Act 1998.

All rights reserved. No reproduction, copy or transmission of this publication may be made without express prior written permission. No paragraph of this publication may be reproduced, copied or transmitted except with express prior written permission or in accordance with the provisions of the Copyright Act 1956 (as amended). Any person who commits any unauthorised act in relation to this publication may be liable to criminal prosecution and civil claims for damage.

Although every effort has been made to ensure the accuracy of the information contained in this book, as of the date of publication, nothing herein should be construed as giving advice. The opinions expressed herein are those of the author and not of MX Publishing.

Paperback ISBN 9781780922034
ePub ISBN 9781780922041
PDF ISBN 9781780922058

Published in the UK by MX Publishing
335 Princess Park Manor, Royal Drive,
London, N11 3GX
www.mxpublishing.co.uk

Cover Design by Staunch Design
www.staunch.com

To our loving parents, Antonia Caro and Janos Zuggo, who bathed us in unconditional love, allowing us to grow.
To our darling husbands, John and Giorgio, who have always been there for us.
To our children, Jasmine and Nicholas, Jonathan and Christopher, whom we love very much, unconditionally.
To our pet dogs, Teddy and Cleo.
This book is written with you in mind, dear reader. We send our love out to you and hope that you will feel it, as you read Entrancing Tales for Change.

Contents

Introduction	9
Butter	12
Lucidota the Glow Worm	13
Make It Happen	15
If You Know	16
The Baby Centipede	17
Overnight	18
Change the Way You Bake a Cake	19
How to Be Your Best You	20
Take Care of Your Feet	21
Salty Tears That Heal	22
A Hug	23
The Donkey Scratched His Beard	24
The Happy Box	25
Horses	26
Nurture Your Thoughts	27
The Rock	28
The Baby Animal	29
Fear of Failure	30
The Shell	31
The White Sofa	32
A Different Street	33
A Conversation with a 92-Year-Old Man	34
The Electric Fence	35
Reflect on Your Successes	36
A Blue Wooden Bench	37
Thoughts Across the Ocean	38
Plasticine Thoughts	39
Olives	40
First Times	41
High Definition	42
Kind Eyes	43

Natural	44
All Roads Lead to Rome	45
Empathic Listening	46
Highlights	47
Kind and Happy Words	48
Wisdom	49
Places to Go	50
A Doctor's Surgery	51
The Painter	52
The You That You Are Now	53
The Hopi Tribe	54
New Friends	55
Together	56
Twenty-One Days	57
Wild Fire	58
Compost	59
Nurture New Ideas	60
Tick Tock	61
Look Into Your Eyes	62
Five Years From Now	63
Acting	64
Free Time	65
Laugh	66
You Can Teach an Old Dog New Tricks	67
The Crystal Palace	68
Changing Patterns in Your Mind	69
A Personal Diary	70
Creams, Potions and Lotions	71
Lavender	72
Simultaneously	73
Between You and You	74
Eggshells	75
Set Your Mind to It	76
Rest Your Mind	77

A Thousand Words	78
The Staircase	79
It's Not Every Day	80
Doors	81
Open Your Mind	82
Italian Minestrone	83
The Right Tools	84
The Resilient Daisy	85
Every Little Bit Helps	86
Friendly Enemies	87
A Hot Shower	88
Healing Wounds	89
On the Loo	90
The Hose Pipe	91
Clothes That Make You Feel Good	92
Just Right	94
The Man Who Lived on the Hill	95
The Dancers	97
Doodling Your Wishes	98
The Same Road	99
Tom	101
Reflections	103
Making Plans	104
Email	106
A Tale of Change	107
Promise Yourself	108
A White Butterfly	109
The Small Pleasures	110
Arrivederci	111
Books That Have Inspired Us	112
About the Authors	113

Introduction

Change is something,
we all know about,
something we all do,
every day,
from the moment we take
our very first breath;
to this moment,
breathing in and out,
right now,
and yet so many find it so hard
to change
something about themselves
that they are not happy with,
and that is a mystery.

The key lies in uncovering
your true self,
digging deep within
to a time
when change
is something you do with ease,
as you change your skin,
without even realising it –
happening all by itself.

As you read this book,
we would like you to
keep in mind
the changes that you
wish to make,

and the steps you
wish to take,
to become a happier
and more successful you,
remembering that
you don't have to do
much at all,
because you are
changing all the time,
like a river is never the same,
and nor are you.
Sometimes,
water can stagnate,
and sometimes thoughts can
twirl and spiral out of control.
However, a river,
knows where to flow,
and so do you,
once you have made
up your mind
to allow your thoughts
to glow.
Change the thoughts
in your mind,
and your mind will
breathe new life.
"Easier said than done," you say.
That's right.
To change your thoughts,
you have to change your mind,
and think new thoughts,
like a plant has to produce new cells,
in order to grow.

You may, at first, find it hard,

but as you read,
you'll find that time is on your side.
A butterfly lives only for a day or two,
and yet, fulfills its due.

As you are reading,
changes are taking place:
your heartbeat slows,
and you displace those thoughts
that you no longer need,
to leave space for new and exciting projects to flow.

Close your eyes, and go inside,
and concentrate on your feet,
and the flow of life
that runs from the soles of your feet,
to the tip of your head.
Allow for feelings to flow
through your body;
allow feelings you no longer need
to leave and float away.
Notice how light, you start to feel,
and notice a smile start to reveal,
deep from within,
changes, are taking place,
healing and soothing,
bathing you now in GLOW.

Butter

Have you ever noticed
what happens to butter
if you leave it uncovered in the fridge?
It appears normal on the outside.
However, when you taste it,
it no longer tastes the same.
If left long enough,
it will absorb any strong odour
coming from other foods close by.
In very much the same way,
your mind will also absorb,
just like butter,
many strong influences
coming your way.
You may enjoy butter
with different flavours
very much.
They may indeed
add an extra touch,
but then again,
you may also prefer
to cover your butter
and to keep it tasting like butter,
pure and simple,
just as it is.
The choice is yours.

Lucidota the Glow Worm

Lucidota was a diurnal glow worm
who lived beneath a tall tree
in a tropical land far, far away.
She spent her time looking for food
during the day and resting at night.
She was a glow worm that did not glow,
but then again that was normal
for a diurnal glow worm,
for they only fly when the Sun is high.
She had heard stories about glow worms
that had a strange light within them,
but it was believed to be nothing more
than a fairy tale.

When the Sun went down,
Lucidota would close her eyes
and fall into a deep sleep,
like all the other diurnal glow worms.
This happened every night -
every night, except for one.
It was a warm summer's night
when Lucidota had the most incredible dream:
she dreamt that she was getting ready to go out,
as she did every day,
only it was not day and the Sun was not high.
It was night.
Pure darkness surrounded her, yet she felt no fear.
Instead, she felt a strange feeling
of excitement and anticipation
as she went out into the night
and headed towards the river.

Along the way, she looked up
into the dark sky and noticed
a glowing light
that grew brighter and brighter.
As she flew closer,
she became aware that it
was being produced by thousands of glow worms,
just like herself.
They were celebrating life itself
and were all glowing in unison.
Very soon, she too was inside
the glow;
she felt a warm energy
that spread all over her body,
and as she looked down,
she noticed that she too glowed.
Upon awakening,
Lucidota told the other diurnal glow worms
about her strange dream
and as she spoke,
she began to glow.
"If she can glow, we can too," they thought,
and so they closed their eyes
and without having to do
anything at all,
they too began to glow,
because that was really how it was meant to be.

Now, they are all diurnal glow worms
that glow
during the daylight hours,
illuminating the shady areas
beneath the tall trees,
there for anyone to see,
because seeing is believing, or maybe not.

Make It Happen

Make it happen today, all by itself.
No need to do much at all - simply glow.
Make it happen by thinking
different thoughts
to those everyday thoughts
that normally climb into your mind.
Climb out of those thoughts
by generating new and exciting
thoughts that take you where you want to go,
without doing much at all,
simply by thinking new and exciting thoughts.
"Don't know how," we hear you say.
Well, simply think of anything but your usual thoughts;
close your eyes,
free up your mind
with a splash of white and dream a dream of change.
What would you like to change?
"Don't know," we hear you say.
Well, that's a good place to start.
Go back and think of what makes you smile,
go back and think of what gives you the get up and go,
make new, exciting and colourful pictures in your mind,
just for pure indulgence.
Forget everything else; these are moments for you.
Live the moment
as you indulge in your new thoughts,
for the moment, and whenever you need to,
you can keep your old thoughts
safely in a corner
and allow these new, exciting and beautiful thoughts and
pictures to come to mind.
What can you imagine?

If You Know

If you know now how to change
by thinking different thoughts,
make it more precise and target your change
in the way you think best.
It's a natural process,
like swallowing or breathing,
to know where you want to go.
Simply take a deep breath and close your eyes;
before long, you will see the light.
The correct way to view where you want to be
is right there inside you.
Take another deep breath
and breathe in the change
as you visualise where you are going
and how you want to be six months from now,
or even a month from now.
If you wish to chunk down,
keep those thoughts
in your mind and believe in yourself,
because we are telling you now
that deep down inside you,
you have all the resources
you need to change.
Only you know how and what to do first,
right now,
to make that change happen for you.
When you open your eyes,
take all the time that you
need to realise how much
you already know
and become aware of the fact
that you may have already begun to change.

The Baby Centipede

The baby centipede had lost its way.
Concrete surrounded its feet.
It looked left and right and not a leaf in sight.
That's not right.
It plodded on,
circled round and round a few times,
and then it stopped fast in its tracks.
That's not right.
Instead of moving backwards
or forwards, it stayed still,
contemplating its next step
or should we say, "steps".
It lay still for what seemed
like a very long time,
dead in its tracks but very much alive,
thinking and thinking
about how to get back
on track without doing anything at all.
Lying there still - ever so still.
Time passed and then
the baby centipede made its move,
just like a chess player ready for a win.
It geared left and then right
and it was back on track
as it headed straight for a piece
of wild grass,
with a thousand shades of green.
As soon as its feet touched
the soft grass, it knew it was home at last
and was glad that
it hadn't done much at all.

Overnight

Overnight, many changes
occur inside your body,
all by themselves,
that you may or may not be fully aware of.
As you gently place
your head upon your pillow
and close your eyes,
your body prepares itself
for the most amazing restoration.
Your cells divide,
tissue synthesises and
growth hormones are released.
All the while, your heartbeat slows down
and your breathing follows,
as you drift off into a comfortable sleep.
The night progresses
and your unconscious mind
provides you with a gift:
you dream whether you are aware of it or not,
and as you dream,
your unconscious mind
processes important information
for you.
All of these changes occur overnight,
while you sleep comfortably,
without having to do anything at all,
allowing you to wake up
feeling refreshed and ready to go.

Change the Way You Bake a Cake

A cake can be baked
in many ways,
as you may well know.
What's stopping you from getting
creative and changing
the way you do it?
If you always follow a recipe,
you'll always get
the same result
and that can be good or not so good,
depending on what you desire.
A splash of extra flour
or extra milk
can make your cake
harder or softer.
A little extra butter
or butter replaced by oil
can change the way your cake tastes.
You can make your cake
lighter and less fattening
or heavier and richer;
the choice is yours,
when you have the courage
to change and experiment
with the way in which
you bake a cake.
You will taste
new flavours in more
ways than one.

How to Be Your Best You

ur tracks and think of all
ings you have done in the past
all the things you're good at.
Think of all the different things you are doing now
and of those you would like to be doing
in the future - why not even tomorrow?
Take a pen and paper and write down
all the things you are good at.
It's curious to notice how
we all have so many resources
and are good at so many things.
You are by no means an exception.
Once you have finished,
take a deep breath
and visualise yourself at your best.
What would you say to yourself?
What would you hear others saying to you?
What would you like to see?
How would you like your best you to be feeling?
What would you be doing?
Who would you be with?
Take all the time you need to ponder,
until you start to notice a change within.
This might not happen
straight away… not now,
but later on,
every time you breathe in deeply
and feel the power
to change within…
tonight and in the days ahead.

Take Care of Your Feet

Take care of your feet,
because putting one foot in front
of the other will take you places.
Take a little time each day
to think about how your feet
are rooted to the ground
and how, when you take
a baby step,
change starts to happen all around.
Consequently, you may choose
to bathe your feet
in good feelings every day
and thank them
for the weight they have
carried today.
Why not make their job
a little lighter and happier
by taking care of where you're going?
It's curious to notice how they'll
thank you back,
by knowing in which direction
you must go.
As you look up towards the heights
you wish to reach,
you may realise
that walking in the right direction
is actually bliss,
because there's nothing stopping you
from moving forward when your feet
and mind work as one.

Salty Tears That Heal

Salty tears
heal internal wounds,
sealing cracks
and making crystals
in your mind,
allowing changes to
occur at deeper levels
than before,
healing,
sealing,
making sure
that you are safe and sound
from now on.
This is your gift
that they leave behind:
a stronger you
that shines
with a thousand crystals
in your mind,
allowing positive
change to happen
all the time.

A Hug

In order to allow
positive change to happen
all by itself,
one of the ingredients that
you need is a hug.
Imagine you
are hugging yourself
from the outside in.
All too often,
you may find that this
is not how you treat yourself
and that's ok because
now you know how to change.
Hug yourself every day
from the outside in.
If you happen to hear
your inner voice
say something
nasty to you,
let it go
and replace it with a hug.
Hugs are very powerful
and not to be underestimated.
Since you now know
how important hugs are,
you can spread the hugs around.

The Donkey Scratched His Beard

The donkey scratched his beard.
This may seem like a funny thing to see in writing,
but the picture that pops into mind can be even funnier.
Our minds are incredible, aren't they?
They produce pictures all day long;
some are funny,
some not so funny, all day long.
All it takes is a thought and off we go,
viewing our own personal film.
It's no wonder that some of us are happy
while others are not.
It's all about what kind of images
are popping into your mind.
Have you noticed how quickly your mood can change
simply by watching a film on TV?
You might start off feeling sad
and end up laughing your head off.
That is a funny expression, isn't it?
'To laugh your head off'.
You laugh and as you laugh,
you laugh off the thoughts that were in your head
prior to watching the film.
It's curious to notice
how powerful our minds really are.
As you become curious about that,
you can also think about how great it is
to be able to have your own personal remote control,
enabling you to change your own
internal states and moods,
simply by changing your thoughts
and maybe even just by thinking
about a donkey who scratches his beard and laughs.

The Happy Box

Childhood memories
come constantly back
with a smell, a thought,
a scent, or a picture,
or maybe even whilst
watching a movie on TV.
Some are happy
and worth keeping safe and sound;
others that make you feel bad,
you can now choose
to let them go.
Feel free to acknowledge
that they may have had a meaning at the time
or served a purpose,
then let go as you breathe out.
Often, memories from
the past can haunt us and hold us back.
Release the emotions
attached to these memories,
especially for the ones you no longer need,
and let them go with the wind.
Create a happy box in your mind
where you can store
all your happy memories.
When you feel the need to smile or laugh,
pull one out and take
a moment to enjoy it as a wonderful gift,
as you move forwards
and create new memories
that will be special to you.

Horses

Wake up to the sound of horses
and hooves galloping in the field,
set free after a night in the stables.
Hear the joy in their gallop
as they explore
the ground beneath their feet.
New ideas flow
as they circle the pine trees.
Watch the power in their bodies
as they tone and keep fit,
simply by doing daily exercise
that is a joy to witness.
They live in the moment
and that can be seen.
In touch with nature,
they scream out their joy
with playful neighs,
whilst they enjoy the morning sun
and smell the mint
and wild herbs in the grass.
They can see life for what it is.
They can sense what they need
and know what to do,
because they can hear the others too,
encouraging them
to enjoy each day blinker-free.
Enjoy your day today;
notice things you may have
not noticed,
like a horse set free to gallop.
That's right:
it's your right to be like that.

Nurture Your Thoughts

You are what you think you are.
If you think that you are great,
you will do great things.
If you think the opposite,
you will be the opposite.
Nurture your thoughts today,
as much as you would
a garden that has been abandoned for
a long time.
Full of brambles and weeds,
it needs delicate and tough
care to put it back into shape.
Think of your thoughts
like the plants in your garden:
uproot the ones that are ruining
the effect you desire
and nurture the ones
that will grow into beautiful plants.
Water them every day
and make sure that they
have good soil,
because that's all they need
to blossom:
water and good soil.
Just as your mind needs quality thoughts,
so does a garden need care and attention.
In order to think quality thoughts,
you have to access them,
either by thinking about things that make you smile,
or by creating new and happy experiences,
by doing and learning something new
that makes you happy now.

The Rock

We would like to tell you a tale
about a rock that lived on a mountain top.
It was surrounded by the most amazing beauty.
One could say it was the luckiest rock in the world,
yet the rock was always too busy being a rock
to notice all the beauty that surrounded it.
This is a shame,
because if it had noticed the beauty,
it might have also taken the time
to become curious about what it had inside.
Deep down inside the rock,
grew a tiny and precious crystal -
a gem if you like,
waiting to be discovered.
This little crystal continued to grow
inside the rock
and waited patiently for the rock
to become aware
of what it had deep down inside.
Sometimes the little crystal
would talk to the rock
when it slept soundly at night
and would tell it about
the wonderful things it had inside.
If only the rock would take the time to notice,
but it could not hear what the crystal had to say
and so carried on day after day,
living its life like a rock,
unaware of the little crystal inside
and of the inner power it could
have access to,
if only it knew how to listen.

The Baby Animal

The newborn baby animal stared at his mum with tender love.
He knew he was on a journey -
a journey called life -
not because he could remember,
but because it was innate in his genes.
As the baby grew, day by day,
he observed his mother's behavior with tender love.
He explored the terrain around him,
sometimes getting into trouble when he would
dare to venture out of his natural boundaries,
soon to be brought back by his mother with a gentle nudge.
All was well, until one day the animal lost his confidence,
not knowing what to do, for he was no longer a baby.
He was an adult like you and me.
He searched high and low for guidance,
finding none until he realised there was
a natural guidance within himself,
ready to know what to do.
So he lay still and displaced all other thoughts.
He felt his feet firmly on the ground beneath him;
he thought about his legs, his body, his arms and knees.
He thought about his breathing happening all by itself
and he knew now, once again,
that the solution was in his mind.
To gain confidence, he just had to imagine himself
doing the things he wanted to do successfully.
That's all.
Like the river next to his field was flowing downstream,
so would new ideas, confidence and inspiration for change
flow, with no trouble at all.
That's when the animal realised it was just like you.

Fear of Failure

She wanted to do it,
but something was holding her back.
It was something so strong
that always knocked her back.
She had new ideas
and could see her big picture
and then her fears kicked in.
Like a kick in the teeth,
they would put her in her place.
Who was she to think that she could
do something so out of reach?
And yet her new ideas kept popping
into her mind
and she would tell her friends and family
about them, hoping for a way out.
And yet all she would get back was a slap in the face.
"That's not for you or us," her family cried.
"How could that idea have even come to your mind?"
Fear held her back and she respected fear,
knowing that if she broke free,
things would change.
Yet somehow, she knew
deep down inside her unconscious mind
that the only way,
for her to be herself,
was to fight fear by taking action
and living her dreams.
That way, she could not fail,
only succeed by learning
from every tiny failure and mistake.
All this gave her new-found confidence,
determination and an inner smile.
Right now!

The Shell

You may have,
at some time or other,
been to the sea.
As you sat on the beach,
you may have found
yourself picking up a shell
and bringing it close
to your ear,
to listen to the sound of the sea.
You may have then
taken it home with you
and put it on a shelf
for many years.
Then, one day for no reason at all,
you happen to pick it up
once again
and bring it close to your ear,
and there it is again:
the sound of the sea.
It's still as clear as
the very first time
you listened.
Time has not changed it at all.

The White Sofa

"Hello,"
said the white sofa.
"It's coffee time;
hope you don't sit on me.
I'm so new and white
and a small stain will
ruin my night.
Please don't sit on me."
So the white sofa
got lucky that night,
because the lady with
the coffee stayed away
and sat opposite on a black chair.
"Phew, that's alright."
Time passed and, more
often than not, the white sofa
was left alone.
So pure and white,
until one night
a furniture van
came to the door
and took the white sofa away.
The white sofa,
stuck in the van,
wished that it had been
more carefree,
knowing now,
that no one would sit on it again.

A Different Street

We don't know how
you usually get home -
whether you take the
train, the Tube, a bus,
or walk, but you do know
your way home.
While on your way
home tonight,
take a different street
to the one you are used to taking.
Look up at the roof tops
and notice what's around you.
You may or may not enjoy
this new route.
One thing's for sure:
you will have changed your ways.
On your way home, you
will have seen something
new or maybe old,
perhaps something you have
not seen in a long time,
simply by taking a different street,
homeward bound.
This gives you a one-way ticket
to successful thinking,
by changing old patterns.

A Conversation With a 92-Year-Old Man

There he was, sitting outside,
under a giant oak tree, at a table next to ours,
in a restaurant up in the mountains,
with the most incredible view.
He smiled and nodded,
as we sat down with our families and friends.
The food was delicious, as we had imagined it to be.
During the meal, he looked over at us several times
and seemed pleased to see that we were enjoying our food.
It was only towards the end of the meal,
when the fresh fruit was served,
that he took the floor and proudly said:
"These peaches are from my peach tree, I'm 92 years old,"
followed by a toothless smile.
He looked so much younger and clearly wanted to talk.
We were impressed, so we asked him:
"Tell us: what's your secret for living such a long life?"
"Well," he answered with an amused look on his face,
"I eat lots of tomatoes, which I grow myself.
If I really want to do something, I go ahead and do it.
I have been criticised by many people,
who are now no longer alive.
The only regret I have is that I never went to the
village dances.
My wife always wanted to go but I never took her."
He then picked up a ripe peach and began peeling it,
with extreme precision and care.
He cut it up into small pieces, put it into a wine glass,
added a little white wine and ate his fruit.
When he finished, he got up slowly,
said, "Arrivederci," and told us that he was making plans
to go on a few trips and do a little sightseeing,
as there was still so much he wanted to see.

The Electric Fence

Electric fences
are put up by horse owners
to keep their
horses
enclosed,
and that is something
that most of you know.
What you
may, perhaps,
not know
is that after a certain
amount of time,
perhaps a year
or maybe two,
when that electric fence
breaks and is no longer of use,
the horse owner
can remove the fence,
and rest assured,
because he knows
that his horses
will not escape.
In their minds, they can see
the fence,
and will not run free.

Reflect on Your Successes

Running through the jungle,
knowing what to cut back,
is an innate art that
we all know how to do,
and that dates back
a long time.
As you begin to map out
your journey,
remember to live life
at the stopovers,
as often,
if not always,
that's where all the action
takes place.
If you're not careful, you
may become aware that
a lifetime of doing has
passed you by,
leaving you unawares.
So, whether it's been ten
or twenty years,
next time,
a moment passes by,
take
the time to enjoy it
for what it is
and reflect
on your successes so far.

A Blue Wooden Bench

Faded blues
and greens come to mind,
as we think of a bench
in the park.
An old wooden oak bench,
stained by the sky and the grass.
So many veins in its body,
all running
in the right direction.
Stories to tell of the people
that have polished it with
loving care,
simply by sitting
there,
telling their story,
to the sky, the grass,
the trees, the passers-by.
Lessons in life,
all on a blue bench
in the park.

Thoughts Across the Ocean

Thoughts across
the ocean,
sweeping waves
of change,
coming in and out
with the ocean spray.
Sending waves of inspiration
all the way to their destination
and only you can tell what
the message is.
Dry your tears and send
them back to sea,
because they
have almost finished
healing you,
as you realise that
what was once yours
no longer
belongs to you,
but to the wind
and the sea.

Plasticine Thoughts

Playing with Plasticine
as a child,
you may have
found yourself forming
lots of different shapes,
because
you knew that
if you made a mistake,
you could
scrunch
it all back up into a ball.
Thoughts are like Plasticine:
as they come
into your mind,
you can take the good ones
and form something new,
something that is flexible
yet durable,
that allows you
to move
in many different ways,
or you can
simply roll them up
into a ball,
and start over again.

Olives

Sunshine making
olives ripen,
in the winter sky,
knowing that a day
of rain will do no harm.
Ladies with wrinkled skin
and happy faces,
smiling
as they harvest
olives one by one by hand.
Their nets catch the fallen
olives nicely, underneath
the trees
rooted there for generations,
and yet experiencing
a new and abundant
crop each year.
Autumn turns to winter
and the Sun continues to shine –
cosmic coloured rays
that lead the way.

First Times

Babies come to mind,
experiencing
new sensations
and first times,
almost every day.
Keep them in mind
as you too have
a first time almost every day.

High Definition

From the low
he climbed to the high,
in one fell swoop.
Once he had read
that he had a choice,
free to choose
high or low.
"I choose high like
the sunshine flies
above the clouds
and is always in
high definition."

Kind Eyes

Photographs can seem
no good
when first seen with
the naked eye
too set on criticizing -
so easy to delete.
Photos get taken
and then discarded
straightaway.
A hair out of place,
a smile that is anything
but pure white -
harsh judging eyes
make the cut as the
photo of oneself is no more.
Kind eyes are needed,
those of a sweet and loving
friend, to view them
with the respect and love
they deserve,
seeing captured in them
moments and emotions
hat filter through
the pictures.
Photos to be kept, treasured
and viewed with kind eyes
forevermore.

Natural

Natural as the wind
blowing in the trees,
natural as your in-breath,
as you breathe in deeply.
Natural as a cup of tea,
as it warms the inside
of your body
and reaches
those parts of you
that need it most.
Some say that nature
knows best:
when to rise,
and when to weep.
There are times when we
may feel sad,
yet the part of us
that is pure nature
knows when to rise
and that is so comforting,
to know that
we really don't have
to do much at all.
Simply look up
at the Moon
and the stars, and remember
that we too
are made of stardust.

All Roads Lead to Rome

People say that all
roads lead to Rome.
So, as you walk along
your road today,
we would like you
to take the time
to wonder,
just a little,
about all those who
have taken your very
same path.
You can become curious
about who those
people were,
about what kind
of lives
they lived,
knowing that you too
will find your way.

Empathic Listening

To be understood
is what everybody needs,
for it is only when
you feel understood,
that you can truly enjoy
what you have
and what you do.
In order to
be understood,
you must first understand
how to listen.
Listening can come
in many different forms.
You can pretend
to listen,
you can ignore
whilst listening,
or you can
become attentive
and listen,
with your eyes
and your heart -
the greatest ears of all:
the empathic kind.

Highlights

As you go about
your day today,
highlight everything
with a highlighting pen.
Just an idea.
Highlight your blues
in blue
and highs
in yellow.
Notice
with curiosity
how balanced
your picture is.
Just an idea.
What colour
would you like
to see and experience
tomorrow?
Make it happen for you.

Kind and Happy Words

Words changing
the way we breathe
and the way we think.
Breathe in deeply.
Think deep,
deep as the
purest water,
where you
can see the bottom
and where you can see
the top and where
you know
that any words
that you pronounce
will drop in deep,
deep into your mind,
for you to keep
or not to keep.
Choose your words
with care today,
bearing in mind
how deep and high,
kind happy words
can take you.
Now.

Wisdom

When we were little,
we used to believe
that old
equalled wise.
Now,
as time has passed,
we have come to see
that he who is old,
is not necessarily wise.
For, at times,
a lifetime
of knowledge
can teach
very little indeed,
because knowing without
wondering
is like
a tree with no leaves.
There are some
who are still very young,
who know so little
and yet they wonder and
ponder about the little
they know
and their curiosity grows.
Those are the ones
whom we call
the wise at heart.

Places to Go

There are places
to go
and visit in one's
mind,
every day,
that will give
you a break
and make you feel
good.
Simply close your
eyes now,
and go inside,
now.
Think of
something or someplace
that makes you
smile
and relax.
Take a moment
to feel and hear
the change in your
breathing, slowing down
now,
ever so deeply,
as you enjoy
the moment
and the place
you've chosen to go to.
Go to it
whenever you
feel the need.

A Doctor's Surgery

A desk,
a chair,
a doctor's glare
and a scare.
Only you know
how to change;
only you know
how to heal.
A doctor
can give you advice,
medicines and help
you on your way.
Remember that only you know
how you feel
and how you are feeling
right now.
Gut feelings and
feeling instinctive
can help you
heal sooner
than you may think.
So remember, the best doctor
in the world cannot
experience what is
inside your body,
because
only you know
that and only you can
reclaim what's
rightfully yours:
the right to know
what's right inside
you all the time.

The Painter

The painter arrived
at seven,
ready to paint
his picture.
All different
colours
could be found
in his mind,
as he stirred
the paint with
the greatest of ease,
making life ever
so easy.
He changed
his mind
and then moved
on to paint
a picture
using his emotions.
It wasn't long
before his
work was almost
done,
but never
to be completed
as he was enjoying
just painting...

The You That You Are Now

"Is that me?"
you say to yourself,
as you happen
to stumble
upon an old photograph,
but then you take
a good look
and see that it is you,
only a different you,
of a long time ago.
It's a you that had different
tastes in food
and clothes,
who knew nothing
about what you do now.
It would be curious
to know
what the other you
in the photograph
would think
about the
you that you are now –
a you,
that has now
changed,
evolved and grown.

The Hopi Tribe

We once read about
a small ethnic group -
a tribe called the Hopi tribe,
who believe that their thoughts travel
and reach those they are directed to.
If a member of the tribe is ill,
the tribe will gather around
and think healthy thoughts,
believing that if
energy is expended,
effects will be produced.
For the Hopi tribe,
thought alone is a
force of energy,
influencing not only one's self
but others too,
and nature itself.
If they think good thoughts
of a healthy growing crop, they believe
the crop will receive these thoughts,
flourish and grow.
This may seem
a little odd and a little strange,
coming from a place that believes
that thought alone
cannot change or modify the world.
Nevertheless, if you take
a moment to think
about the Hopi tribe,
it becomes natural to believe
that thought
does indeed leave traces
everywhere it goes.

New Friends

The world is full of people,
all around us,
and yet so many of us are lonely.
Take a look around you
as you take a walk
and as you go about your business tomorrow.
Notice all the faces -
some happier than others -
and wonder how many lonely people are simply
waiting for a smile, a word, a gesture of humanity.
At the gym and in town, notice all the people
around you and open up to the
possibility of making a new friend today,
because an extra word, an extra smile,
a handshake and a "Pleased to meet you"
set the scene and break the ice,
allowing new friendships to be born.
All the lonely people in this
world today
need a little help from you.
Give out an extra smile
and introduce yourself,
chat or have a cup of tea or coffee together.
Sow the seeds of friendship
and reap the rewards.
Who will benefit more from this
new relationship:
you or them?
Lonely no more.

Together

The conscious and unconscious
minds together.
One mind thinking, one mind feeling –
a perfect balance,
like day and night
or the Sun and the Moon.
You may already
be aware of the fact
that it is
your unconscious mind
that does the feeling,
the dreaming
and all things that
occur automatically
inside you.
That can be
so comforting to know.
It would be so difficult
to have
to think consciously
about blinking
before you
blink,
wouldn't it?

Twenty-One Days

Daily habits are hard
to break at first,
without the right mindset.
With the right mindset
held in your mind,
they become as easy
as can be.
It takes twenty-one days
to create a new habit
or routine,
so when experiencing
some sort of change
in your life,
make sure
you give it twenty-one days
to see if it's right for you.
Twenty-one days
can make
all the difference.
Remember that.

Wild Fire

Flames high in the sky
of a fire out of control.
Thoughts in your mind
spiralling out of control.
Wild and negative thought
processes are so hard to
control when you
are unaware
that they
are like a fire that
has been left to its own
devices,
without the
boundaries that it merits
and needs.
All it needs,
like those thoughts,
is a hose and some water.
Now,
where the ashes
simmer on the ground,
new and fertile thoughts
of positive new beginnings
start to sprout...

Compost

The compost heap
at the bottom of the
garden, behind some trees,
looks pretty lifeless,
piled full of dead leaves,
cut grass and flower heads,
long dried
out by the midday sun.
Spilling over and out
into the flowerbeds,
what looks so chaotic is,
in fact,
in perfect balance with nature
and brimming
with life.
All it takes for
new seedlings
to sprout is a few months,
some rain
and some extraordinary time.
Before long,
what was once dried and dead
is reborn
and becomes new earth -
compost full of nutrients,
to sustain new life,
full of seedlings
ready to sprout
in the ground
and in your mind.

Nurture New Ideas

New ideas
in your mind
can disappear
as soon as they've arrived,
if not nurtured
with loving care,
if not protected
from the publics glare.
Nurture your idea
as you would a new seedling,
covering it with cotton wool,
until it has the strength
to carry on all by itself.
Water it and feed it
every day,
until one day
you see that it has
grown and gained
momentum,
all by itself.
It no longer needs
you hands-on
all of the time,
only the necessary
amount of time to see it
flourish and prosper.

Tick Tock

Tick tock
goes the clock.
As you listen to its sound
and steady rhythm,
you start
to fall asleep.
You start
to close your eyes
and start
to slow
your breath,
and as you slow
your in-breath,
and your out-breath
deepens,
those new ideas
that you have nurtured
start to grow
in your mind.
You dream
of what they will become
and only you know
how and when
the tick tock
of the clock
will reveal your
true potential, now
in the making.
While you sleep,
the tick tock
of the clock
is there making
your possibilities come true.

Look Into Your Eyes

The mirror
sees a thousand eyes,
daring to stare.
You look into
the mirror
and see
a thousand eyes
glare back at you.
Look into
your eyes with
intent to see
what's there.
See and desire
what you wish for
and see what you'd
like to stay the same,
knowing all the while,
that a thousand eyes
are better than two.
Look around
in all directions
and dimensions,
and keep your
mind open to
what you
see
your eyes saying
to you,
from the mirror
on the wall.

Five Years from Now

Five years from today,
where will you be?
What will you be doing
and what will you see?
Who will you be with
and what will you be like?
It's alright not to know -
nobody knows for sure -
although we know
that it's a good idea
to have an idea
and a dream.
If you don't
know where you're going,
it's harder to get there.
Au contraire - when you do
know where you're going,
things fall
into place easily
and manifest for you,
because once
you are aware of
the road you are travelling on
and know
where you're going,
you'll get there quickly.

Acting

Act the part
and you'll get the part.
Dress for the part
and before long
you'll be playing that role.
Play the role
with passion,
be yourself
and the crowd
will love you.
Own up to your insecurities
and your insecurities
will disappear.
Stand up and speak
of your fears,
and they will
melt away into the distance,
having nothing to
feed off.
Your stage awaits
you now...

Free Time

A little free time
can go a long
long way –
free to be
what you wish to be
and to go where you
wish to go.
Ten minutes,
all to yourself,
are sometimes
all you need.
No television
to get in your way,
no news,
that brings
nothing new
to burden you today,
only free time,
solo,
for you.
Time to look out
of the window
and stare up at a tree,
freeing up
your mind
as you watch
the branches
moving in the wind.

Laugh

There can be times in your life
when you forget how to laugh –
when you forget how easy it is
to let go of that smile
that you keep imprisoned inside.
It doesn't take much at all
to free it all up,
simply a little smile
that doubles up into a laugh.
Laughter is inside you,
there for you to use,
innate and inborn.
You know what it feels
like to have a good laugh -
when you let go
of your self criticisms and doubts.
Weave it into
the fabric of your daily life,
as an expert tailor
would - with care and ease.
For laughter is one of the
little things in life that counts,
big time!

You Can Teach an Old Dog New Tricks

"I don't know
how to do that,"
is something
that we have all said
to ourselves.
We forget how quickly
we could learn,
if only
we allowed
learning
to come into our minds.
We remember to do
the most incredible things,
yet we forget to remember
how to learn new things.
"You can't teach an old
dog new tricks,"
is something
we have all heard before,
misleading us to believe
it was the old dog
that could learn no more.
"You can't teach an old
dog new tricks,"
Is that really true?

The Crystal Palace

There is a place
right between
your eyes,
a special place
often called
the third eye,
home to the pineal gland,
thalamus,
and hypothalamus too.
In Taoism,
it is referred to as
The Crystal Palace -
a place full of energy and light.
This is where
the inner smile is born -
a smile that comes
from within the heart,
liver, kidneys and lungs.
Whether you believe
this to be true or not,
imagine
all your organs in your body
saying, "hello," to each other
and smiling from within.
It is a smile so radiant
that it makes you feel
as if crystals
are shining within you,
giving you an infinite glow.

Changing Patterns in Your Mind

A crowded room,
with lots of clutter,
makes it hard
to see what you really
need and what
you no longer need.
Clear out your rooms
on a regular basis,
preferably every day,
before you go to bed
at night and rest,
restful dreams
of how you want
things to be
from now on,
shiny and clear,
ready
to move towards
your goals.

A Personal Diary

Keep a little 'journey'
of your successes,
logged in a
notebook or diary,
by the side
of your bed.
Register everything that
you wish to do
in your own hand -
whether you write
with your right hand or left
is not important at all.
All that matters
is that you cherish,
what you are grateful for
each day
and make your future plans
for tomorrow.
Watch
how you begin
to grow and change
day by day,
from now on.

Creams, Potions and Lotions

How many creams,
potions and lotions
do we bathe our bodies
in every day?
What about our minds?
How do you bathe
yours everyday?
Do you bathe
yours in luxurious
creams and lotions,
or do you leave it
barren and dry?
Or do you allow
others to fill your mind
with their fears and anxieties,
causing you endless stress?
Detoxify your mind,
from today,
by soothing it,
with luxury creams
and potions,
whilst you enjoy,
laugh and learn
new things.

Lavender

Look into
a row of lavender
and allow
yourself
to experience
it with all your
senses:
the pretty colour,
the gorgeous
scent and how
it feels
as you rip
the flowers off the bud.
Your hands are now
immersed in a
strong scent
of lavender oils,
ready to relax
and strengthen you.

Simultaneously

While we are in the process
of writing this book,
other things and events
are happening simultaneously,
in our lives.
If you take a moment to think about it,
you will notice that
this happens to you too,
all the time.
As you are reading this hypnotic tale,
you are also breathing naturally,
your heart is beating regularly,
and your nails
are growing steadily.
While you sit there comfortably,
wondering
maybe a little
about how fascinating
simultaneous occurrences can be,
you can only begin
to imagine how much information
your unconscious mind
has already begun to absorb,
tale after tale.
We don't know when these occurrences
may take place,
while your conscious mind
is involved in reading these words,
or they may take place
as you walk home from school,
or on your way to work.
This indeed is a comforting thought.

Between You and You

Many things occur between
you and you -
some you are aware of,
others maybe not so.
This may cause conflicting ideas
that create
inner obstacles,
friction and unease.
You see, at times
your conscious mind
may not be in tune
with your unconscious mind,
or subconscious mind,
if you prefer,
and you may have a feeling
that something is not quite right,
or perhaps even a dream late at night,
that is telling you
to change your ways.
Call it a gut feeling or a premonition,
it doesn't really matter.
The important thing
is for you to be in tune with your inner you.
When you are,
when you listen to what
you have to say to yourself,
your conscious mind and your unconscious mind
will be balanced,
balancing you and you.

Eggshells

Cracking an egg open,
eggshells
came to mind:
strong enough
to nurture a chick
with all the resources
needed within,
creating new life,
and yet easily
broken in half.
Resilient and yet
delicate,
a little like your insides.
Treat your delicates
with care,
including your mind,
and the results
will be a super,
natural resilience
like an eggshell
that hasn't
been crushed.

Set Your Mind to It

Set your mind,
much like you
would your alarm clock every night.
Today, set it to do and think
about the things
you wish to carry out tomorrow.
Free up your mind from worry,
as you set your mind
each day and open it up
to new ideas,
knowing that worrying less
or not at all may be a good thing.
All the while,
keep in mind that a
little worry can be a good thing,
needed to address certain
issues or problems
and make you take
the necessary action.
Know that
when you set your mind
each night and allow time
for creativity and for dreaming,
you will be free to dream.
When you dream and plan,
you will find that action
follows soon after and your dreams
become your reality.
It doesn't take long;
trust in you.

Rest Your Mind

Rest your mind
from old habits,
by creating new ones
that inspire,
motivate and generate
creativity in you.
Take a walk
under your favourite
trees in the park.
Ride a bike
like when you were a child.
That takes
you back, doesn't it?
Back to creative times,
when playing
was normal
and role playing was
a part of everyday life.
Bring into today
that child so full
of curiosity
for learning,
so active and such fun.
And if you cannot
recall such a child,
there is always
time now to
act and live
in such a fun-loving way.

A Thousand Words

A thousand words
or maybe only one.
One word
to make you smile.
One word that has
a very special effect on you,
deep down inside.
One word that
can instantly change your mood.
Take a moment
to think about that word
now
and as it comes to mind,
notice
how it makes
you feel,
then say it out loud
so that your outer ears
can hear it too.
Let the sound
of that special word
caress your ears
and then
as it re-enters into you,
once more,
put it in a special place
to treasure forevermore.

The Staircase

A staircase can take
you up
or it can take you down.
Whichever way
you decide to go,
up or down,
will be the right way
for you.
You can,
if you like,
take the time
to appreciate the view
and surprise yourself,
as you become aware,
of the things,
around you
and the thoughts
inside you,
knowing that
you have all the resources
inside you to change
anything you need to change.
That doesn't have
to happen
right now.
It can begin to happen
as soon as you decide
to take your next step
up or down.

It's Not Every Day

It's not every day that you wake up
with an idea in mind –
an idea so powerful,
that you know it will change your world,
an idea that, if you dare
start to execute and put into practice,
will stretch your limits and challenge you,
more than ever before.
Allow this to happen to you,
because we can assure you
it feels ever so good.
When you happen to feel
this kind of force within you,
it takes over
and you become like a bumble bee
going for its nectar.
You may find yourself
fumbling and mumbling
in what seems like the dark,
as you go about your day;
that would be normal.
Above all, you must keep in mind
the honey and the nectar
that belongs to you,
because when you wake up
with an idea in mind,
you are like the honey bee
who will do everything and anything
to produce the honey and have a feast.

Doors

As young children,
we see a door and our brain does a very clever thing.
Once we have learnt what a door looks like,
what a door does, how it opens and closes,
and what it's called, we generalise and our brain can,
from then on, recognise any kind of door.
Quite clever, don't you think?
It's something we usually take for granted.
Just as we use generalisation to tell us what a door
looks like and how to open any kind of door,
we often over-generalise in our lives
and that can sometimes hinder us,
instead of helping us move on.
For instance, Joe was nearly bitten by a dog
when he was young and, from then on,
he made a general statement to himself,
at an unconscious level,
that all dogs were too be feared.
As he got older, he had another bad experience with a dog
and that made him get a dog phobia.
So, generalisation can be a good thing or a bad thing.
Next time you see a door, make sure you realise
that doors open possibilities and opportunities
and the more doors you open as opposed to close,
the more open-minded you will become.

Open Your Mind

As you are reading this tale,
open your mind to the possibility
that you have endless
possibilities within you.
Open your mind to the
fact that you are ready
to mine these possibilities;
reach out and find your gold.
Your gold is the treasure inside of you
that has been hidden under layer
upon layer for so long.
Layer upon layer
lifts as each day
you awake with a new
gift for yourself -
that of an open mind.
Be ready to acknowledge
that, yes, maybe you have made mistakes,
and that's okay.
Be ready to acknowledge
that you have learnt from your mistakes,
now knowing that
as you learn new things and take new steps,
your gold has surfaced,
and surprised you down to your core.
You now realise that it is 24-carat pure
unconditional love,
to share with the world,
making everything else
seem unimportant and alright now.

Italian Minestrone

There are really no limits
as to what ingredients
you can add
to an Italian minestrone soup.
That is something
we have learnt over time.
A little potato, some tomatoes,
a few beans here and there,
maybe a sprinkle of fresh basil,
to give it that delicious taste.
There you have it,
ready to eat and healthy too.
So, as you go about
your day today,
imagine
you are making
an Italian minestrone
and take a little bit of this,
and a little bit of that,
from whatever you can see,
hear and taste,
that takes your fancy.
Put your ingredients
together and give them a stir.
At the end of the day,
you will have
experienced what life
tastes like,
as you enjoy your own
special minestrone soup.

The Right Tools

Try swatting a fly
without a fly swatter.
It can be a difficult task,
taking a long time,
until you may finally give up.
Yet, with a fly-swatter in hand,
that fly can be gone
within a moment or two,
causing you trouble no more.
Try putting a nail in
the wall without a hammer and see
how that goes -
very frustrating indeed.
The right tools can help you get along,
to do things with grace and ease.
Reading this book
will give you the right tools
to make the
right amount of changes
in your life.
It will give
your unconscious mind
the right tools
to get along and fix anything
that needs fixing.
Furthermore,
once you possess
the right tools,
future projects
can be carried out with ease.

The Resilient Daisy

There are times in your life when you can feel tired,
maybe because you have worked too hard,
or maybe because you have worked too little,
as that too can make you feel tired.
Whatever the reasons may be,
we would like you to take a moment
to think about how a daisy lives its life.
If you have the chance to step outside,
you might even get the opportunity
to look at and observe these amazing little flowers.
Some people consider them weeds,
others think they are simply pretty,
but if you look up close,
you will notice how flexible their stems are.
If you happen to step on one,
you will see how it bends down
only to bounce back up within a few seconds or so!
That is indeed an incredible thing,
to have one so heavy step on one so light
and apparently weak.
As you take the time to think about the incredible
resilience that daisies possess,
we would like you to become aware
whenever you are ready -
and that may be now or the next time
you happen to see a daisy -
that you too possess great resilience,
that you too can be flexible enough not to break,
and that you can take great pride in
knowing that you too can bounce back up.
Deep down inside,
you have the flexibility and resilience of a daisy.

Every Little Bit Helps

Little by little,
as you take each new breath,
and slowly breathe in and out,
allow the release of
tension to leave you feeling great…
but not just yet!
Notice how your
feet are firmly on the ground and how,
when you clench your fists as hard as you can,
you can allow the tension in your
jaw to disappear, into thin air.
Little by little and bit by bit,
you feel a warm feeling start to spread
from the centre of your
stomach all the way up to your mind.
As your mind clears,
you start to think.
Think about how
you want to improve your situation,
think about what you could do
if you had no limitations,
think about how it would feel to be this way,
all the while knowing
that today is your day,
for making this happen.
Dare to dream for what you wish for.
As you dream, start to smile,
knowing that tomorrow
will bring you success bit by bit,
as every little bit helps
you on your way.

Friendly Enemies

To hate someone
or dislike a person
can only bring you heartache.
Who is it that suffers
more: your so-called enemy or you?
How do you feel
when you think about this person?
"Not so good," we hear you say.
Where do you feel the anger?
Is it in your mind and in your gut,
as you feel your heart
race and your body begin to shake?
Shake off this feeling
now by stepping out of yourself.
Look at your situation
from somebody else's point of view.
Does this person really
deserve all your heartache?
By distancing yourself
from your enemies
and detaching yourself,
you are finally free to take a
pair of scissors and cut the umbilical cord
that ties you to them.
When you do so, now or in a while,
you will finally be free to move on.

A Hot Shower

A long day at work
can be tiring
to say the least,
although sometimes
inspiring
if you are in,
the right line of work for you.
When you get
home in the evening
or the next morning,
take time in the shower
to relax and recharge.
For, just as plants need water,
you too can
benefit greatly
from being bathed
by the soft sprinkles of a hot shower.
Your muscles
start to relax and unwind
as the water
moisturises and lubricates your mind,
allowing for
new thoughts to enter it and flow.
Like the drops
of water that settle on
your skin,
your mind
becomes open to new suggestions
of well-being,
as you begin to feel ever so relaxed.

Healing Wounds

There may have been times
in your life
when you have fallen down
and maybe bruised your knee,
or accidentally cut yourself.
You probably put a plaster on,
without giving it
much thought at all,
knowing that
your body would heal itself
in its own time,
in maybe a day or two.
We would like you
to take a moment
to think about how this amazing
process occurs.
You can wonder,
if you like,
about how other wounds can heal
in very much the same way,
even though these other
wounds may
not need a plaster,
as they may be
wounds of a different kind.
Give them a little time
and the healing process
will start straightaway.
You can take comfort in this,
as it is true.

On the Loo

The next time you are on the loo
and you reach out for the loo paper,
take a moment to
ponder this:
almost all of us use loo paper.
Of course there are a few exceptions
in the more remote
parts of the world.
However, they too have their
alternatives.
The next time
you feel intimidated by someone,
for whatever reason -
for example, by your boss
or by someone
who seemingly occupies
a very important role in society,
someone you feel
has the power to make
you feel small -
remember the loo paper.
We all use it and
they are no exception,
so let out a giggle
when you see
them next and keep
this thought in mind,
because now you
know for sure that we all use
loo paper and sit on the loo!

The Hose Pipe

Sitting in the garden,
soaking up the Sun,
allowing the rays of sunshine to
work their magic,
lurking amongst the flowerbeds,
lies the hosepipe.
It's a wonderful invention:
a tool that carries water from the tap
to wherever you like,
in such an easy and magical way,
almost like child's play.
It is something so wonderful
and yet something that most
people take for granted.
The hosepipe comes
in many sizes, to
fit every requirement,
and can even be cut to size if so need be,
when bought by the yard or metre.
The water that flows through its insides
can be turned off and on
whenever need be.
It can even be programmed
to come on and switch
off at certain times
throughout the day or night,
all at the flick of a switch –
a real marvel indeed.

Clothes That Make You Feel Good

We all have an outfit in our wardrobe
that makes us feel great when we wear it.
It's the special outfit that we keep
for a special occasion.
It's not too dressy,
but smart enough
to be worn every day
if we so wished.
Yet most of us may find that it
remains in our wardrobe
and is only worn when we want
to look our best.
Here is a suggestion that comes
from a long way back –
from a different era –
and a different country…
from Madrid after the Second World War.
Resources were scarce
and there wasn't much luxury around;
a lady had just one black elegant dress
and a matching black coat,
one pair of good
shoes and matching
black handbag.
This lady would be seen
in elegant circles
always wearing the same thing.
When she dressed like this,
in her Sunday best,
she felt good,
she felt great,
she felt as if she could do

or be anything
and go anywhere
with a smile.
It's not about how much money
you may or you may not have
to buy clothes,
it's about wearing clothes
that make you smile,
that make you feel good
the moment you slip them on.
Whether you are male or female,
dig out your best outfit
and wear it every day.
You will be sure
to notice a difference
in you,
in more ways than one.

Just Right

Water runs within your body,
hydrating and
keeping you alive.
It is the right
amount of water that
you need throughout the day,
every day.
Thirst makes you drink a glass
or two and then some more,
but sometimes you may be out of sync
and have forgotten how to drink
water every day.
Plants in garden pots
droop when they are dry
and you know they need a drink of
water and comply.
Your body is the same
and your skin starts to feel dry.
You may find yourself over-eating,
because you are thirsty
without even realising it.
Keep this in mind
as you go about your day,
because plants
need water to thrive
and you are no different to them,
in body and mind.

The Man Who Lived on the Hill

There are many reasons
why one would choose to live on a hill.
It could be to enjoy the view,
or to breathe in the fresh air,
or simply to be closer to the sky.
We don't know why the man in our story
chose to live on a hill,
but we do know how he passed his time.
His name was Elims -
a difficult name to say without a smile indeed.
If you spell it backwards you'll see what we mean.
Elims was, as he always said himself,
the happiest man on Earth.
He cultivated sunflowers for a living,
which meant that he
was surrounded by seeds, earth and yellow.
Every day, he watched them grow,
and if he watched closely enough,
he could see how they opened and closed.
He called them smileflowers
because of how they made him feel.
Elims quickly realised
that they followed the Sun's path
and would generally face east.
He laughed and said they had a
one-track mind:
all they could think about was sun
and more sun and more sun.
He spent his days walking through
the sunflower fields,
checking that everything

was well.
Every now and again,
he staked a flower
to protect it from the wind,
for his sunflowers
were the giant kind,
which grew up
to three metres tall.
He would maintain
the soil - deep and rich -
which would, in turn,
feed the sunflowers beautifully.
On returning to his house on the hill,
he said to himself that he was
the happiest man on Earth,
because not only was he surrounded
by beauty and joy,
he could also eat the sunflower seeds,
thus enabling the happiness to grow
deep inside him.
That is how Elims lived to a hundred and five.
A life worth living
and a seed worth planting –
the happiness kind.

The Dancers

Have you ever noticed
how dancing makes you feel?
Hear a tune in your head
and feel your body start to move
in tune to the music.
Watch how babies sway to and fro
as they hear the music flood
through their ears and bodies.
Do your daily tasks today
with that extra bounce in your step
and notice how easy
it is to go about your day
from one place to the next,
getting things done.
Some countries across the Atlantic
live on music
that feeds their very existence
and it's as necessary
to them as is the
sunshine that shines
and makes them smile.
Their bodies are
supple and agile
and they know what to eat,
to keep their waist
trim enough to gyrate
in tune to the melodies
that are life itself to them.
They are dancers
from all walks of life,
united in music and love.

Doodling Your Wishes

Take a pen and paper
and start to doodle with intention.
First of all, doodle
whatever comes to mind as your hand
circles the paper.
Then, start to think
about what you wish for
and doodle your wishes on that paper,
in any form that represents them.
Let your hand
be free to flow,
as the pen caresses the paper lightly,
for doodles come
from your unconscious mind
as do your true wishes.
Spend some time on this and make
sure that you have
an abundance of ink and of paper.
Imagine you could wave a magic wand
and you could have
anything and everything you want.
What would you wish for now?
What does your pen doodle now?
Dream freely as you doodle away,
because dreams
that are planned out on paper
have a habit of becoming
reality -
ask any inventor or creator.

The Same Road

June left the house at 7am every morning,
and every morning, she drove down the
same road to get onto the main road.
This road was in a terrible condition,
all full of bumps and holes.
Every time June drove down it,
she would grumble and swear to herself,
wishing that someone would do
something about it.
"It really should be fixed," she would think,
as she drove past,
bouncing all the way down.
One day, June punctured a tyre on
that bumpy road
and that added to her frustration,
but soon after that, there she was again,
bright and early,
driving on that same terrible road.
Her gardener, a wise man,
suggested that she take an alternative route.
To her surprise, this thought had never
even crossed her mind.
He told her about a small side road,
behind her house.
He warned her that it might take a little longer
to reach the main road,
but that she was assured a smooth ride.
June thought about what her gardener had said
and wondered why she had never thought
about changing routes.
On the way to work the next morning, at 7 am,
June gave the smooth new road a passing thought,

but it was just too early to think about change,
and so off she went down that
same bumpy road,
moaning and swearing,
all the way down to the main road.
On her way back from work,
once again her gardener's words
and the smooth new road
came to mind,
but she was far too tired,
after a hard day's work
to think about change and so
she took that
same bumpy road back home,
bouncing up and down once again.

Tom

Tom was reading a book
about change.
He read the last pages and
put the book down.
He thought about
what he had just read:
"You cannot change the whole world
around you,
but you can become
increasingly aware,
day after day,
that the person
you can change is you!"
He had heard that before.
It was nothing new,
yet it provided him
with an immediate sense of relief.
There were often times in his life
when he had wanted others
around him to change.
When he was a kid,
he always wished that
his parents would change.
Now he was all grown up,
he often wished his partner
would change.
Thinking about it now,
he spent a lot of his time
hoping and wishing
for people around him to change,
yet he hadn't thought so much
about changing himself.

He started thinking that maybe
he could change.
Maybe he could change the way
he looked at others.
Maybe he could hear what his partner
had to say
with empathic ears,
as it said in the book,
and really listen.
Maybe he could finally really
listen to himself.
As Tom was thinking
about change,
he looked in the mirror
and smiled,
knowing now that
 his smile
would reach him
deep down inside
and this was just
the beginning.

Reflections

Reflections of how you are acting
and of your behaviour
are all around you, all the time.
Your moods are contagious
and will be caught by those nearby.
Whether you are feeling ratty,
happy or sad,
be aware that those around you
will be influenced.
Know that you have the power
to change the dynamics
around you always.
This may be surprising,
but it's true.
You may wonder why
your children always act up,
why they shout and scream,
or why somebody is taking advantage of you.
In all situations, the first person
to check out is yourself.
That may be hard to believe,
because we all tend
to attribute fault to somebody else.
Change your internal state
of well-being:
talk to the people in your world,
coming from a place of calm confidence.
Add a smile and a lovely word;
watch how your actions are reflected,
almost like looking in the mirror -
a mirror of your emotions,
reflected across your world.

Making Plans

Each new tomorrow
brings with it the opportunity
for you to take a deep breath
and collect your thoughts.
Whilst you do so,
make plans in your mind.
Think them through
and act them out,
step by step and
day by day.
Make sure that each day
brings about a little change.
As each hour ticks by,
do something that will take you
where you want to be,
whether it's thinking
in a new and constructive way
or whether it's
taking a concrete action
that will bring you one
step closer to going where you
want to be.
Do this right now and
in the days and weeks to come.
Remember that plans
can be evaluated and upgraded
as you go along
and that the flexibility
of your mind
is the key to your success.
The branches of a willow tree
bend and sway in the wind,

growing all the time.
They are as supple as your mind is,
now that you have read each tale.
Know all the while
that excitement and enjoyment
will make you grow each day,
in such a happy and delightful way.
All the birds will wish
to rest on your branches
blowing in the wind,
because you have discovered
your inner strength,
also known as
your unconscious mind.

Email

This is a personal tale
of how some people resist change.
They fight it with
every instrument they know,
until they realise it made
sense all along.
Around eighteen years ago,
in an international organisation,
email was being introduced
to take over the old memo system.
The number of people
who complained each day
was mind-blowing.
Nobody wanted the change.
In the same
international organisation today,
emails are the main method
of communication used by the staff,
which just goes to show
how something
that was so contested at the time
is so loved today.
It is reported that
one can hear the complaints
when the email system
has a problem.
A change is as good as a rest.
Remember that.

A Tale of Change

A tale of change begins with a smile.
This tale could be about
you, or you,
because, by the time you have reached
this very page,
many changes have already taken place.
You now know
how heavy some thoughts can be,
and how wonderful
and easy it is to set yourself free.
You may surprise yourself one day.
One day, out of the blue,
you'll say, "That is exactly what I will do."
You may wonder
why you had never thought about it before,
yet deep down inside,
it will feel just right.
You have so much inside you
yet to be discovered,
so many things you can do,
that at first you thought you could not do.
You learnt to
hold a pencil in your hand and write;
you can learn to smile
as changes come your way,
because this is the tale of your life.
As you read and absorb
the meaning of these words,
you can absorb something new.
No regrets.

Promise Yourself

Mother Nature knows best
and so do you.
There can be no disagreement with that.
When you trust your gut instincts,
it's easy to find your way.
It's easy to know
what you love doing and to do it
every day, because that's how
we thrive as human beings.
by doing what we love,
little by little, every single day.
Cultivate a passion,
as you would a garden,
and if you think that's
an impossible task, think again.
You don't have to do it all by yourself;
you can and should ask for help.
Look out for like-minded
people that can offer help and support.
Go back to your books if you have to.
Before long, you will find that your passion
has a drive and momentum of its own.
It's easier and more pleasurable
to do now, then ever before.
And you will be well on your way
to discovering the key
to what makes you smile.
Do what you love doing,
at least for part of your day,
every day and take a moment or two
to feel how powerful and
beautiful that is.

A White Butterfly

Our mother used
to say, upon seeing
a white butterfly,
that, "a letter was
coming in the post."
How many white
butterflies will
fly your way
and how many letters
will you receive today?
How many letters
will you send out
and how many butterflies
will you spot?
Watch out for the meanings
you attach to things,
because sometimes
a white butterfly
is purely and simply that:
a white butterfly to admire,
in all its splendour.

The Small Pleasures

Enjoy the small pleasures
in your day today,
as they may be the greatest
pleasures of all.
The smiles,
the cuddles,
the warm drinks,
your friends,
your couch,
a book to read,
a field of grass,
a park,
a tree,
your pets,
a walk.
Enjoy the small pleasures
in your day because it's
these special moments
that make your life
a great pleasure to live,
each and every day.

Arrivederci

Well, the time has come to say,
"bye-bye," or as they say in Italy,
"arrivederci," which translated literally
means, "until we next meet."
Quite sweet, really, we think.
It's lovely to notice the meaning of words,
in the language we use every day,
because words have a powerful
effect on our nervous system,
and that is something very powerful indeed.
This is a discovery we made a long time ago,
which has changed our lives in many ways.
Words can be our friends or foes.
They can make you feel good or bad, happy or sad,
simply by talking, whether it's out loud
to somebody else, or to yourself.
Choose your words carefully and if by chance
you catch yourself using a word that makes you feel
less than good, make sure to stop it and change it
for a word that offers you new possibilities.
Choose and use your words with care from now on,
as the richer your vocabulary, the more
freedom you possess to express yourself.
Moreover, you will experience your
world in different ways because words spoken
have the power to move mountains inside you,
to make rivers flow in your veins,
to make you quiver or tremble with excitement,
to make you feel like a child,
experiencing language for the first time,
to allow you to glow and shine.
Words change your mind.

Books That Have Inspired Us

Erickson, Milton H. My Voice Will Go With You – The Teaching Tales of Milton H. Erickson. (Rosen Sidney, Editor) W.W Norton & Company, Inc. 1991

Bandler, Richard. Richard Bandler's Guide To Trans-Formation. Deerfield Beach:FL Health Communications, Inc., 2008

Bandler, Richard. Get the Life You Want. Deerfield Beach:FL Health Communications, Inc., 2008

Bandler, Richard and Fitzpatrick Owen. Conversations with Richard Bandler.
Deerfield Beach:FL Health Communications, Inc., 2009

Bandler, Richard and John LaValle. Persuasion Engineering. Cupertino, CA: Meta Publications. 1996

Grinder, John and Bandler, Richard. The Structure of Magic Vol.1 Cupertino, CA: Meta Publications, 1975

Grinder, John and Bandler, Richard. The Structure of Magic Vol.2 Palo Alto: CA: Science and Behaviour Books, 1976

Robbins, Anthony. Awaken The Giant Within: Free Press Simon & Schuster. Inc. 1991

About the Authors

The English Sisters are Violeta and Jutka Zuggo. They were born in London, and now live in sunny Rome with their lovely families. They have always been very close and have often been mistaken for twins. Language has always played a very important role in their lives, as they grew up in a bilingual family. This led to a natural fascination with how language affects the brain.

They are qualified in the Theory and Principles of Indirect Hypnosis, Ericksonian Psychotherapy and NLP, with Stephen Brooks' British Hypnosis Research.
The English Sisters have developed their own personal style of conversational hypnosis, with their 'Hypnotic Ramblings for Change' videos that guide the viewer into a state of light trance, whilst bringing about positive changes. Their videos are appreciated worldwide.

The English Sisters have also developed their own methodology of teaching English to Italians, using NLP and Conversational Ericksonian Hypnosis, on their online English course. It's the first of its kind. They are the authors of 'Don't Learn English, Smile / Non Imparare l'Inglese, Sorridi'.

Websites:
http://www.hypnoramblings.com
http://www.englishsisters.com

Email: englishsisters@gmail.com

Also from MX Publishing

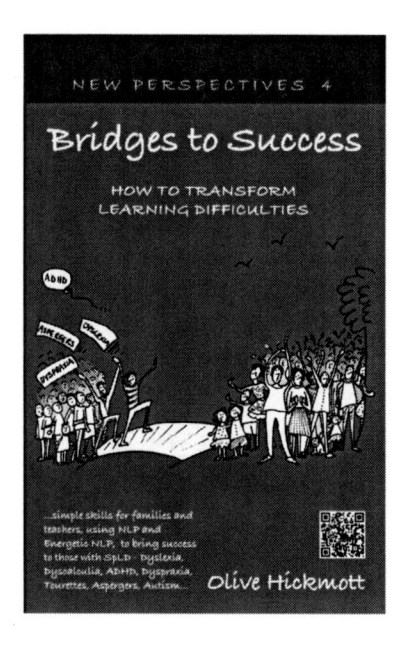

Bridges to Success: Keys to Transforming Learning Difficulties; Simple skills for families and teachers to bring success to those with learning difficulties using NLP and Energetic NLP

Also from MX Publishing

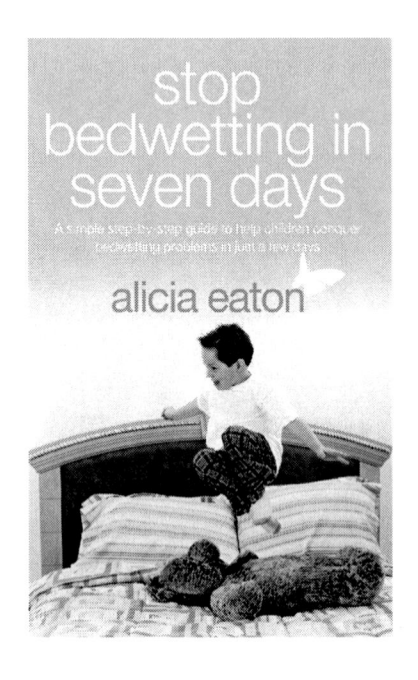

Stop Bedwetting in 7 Days: A simple step-by-step guide to help children conquer bedwetting problems in just a few days

Also from MX Publishing

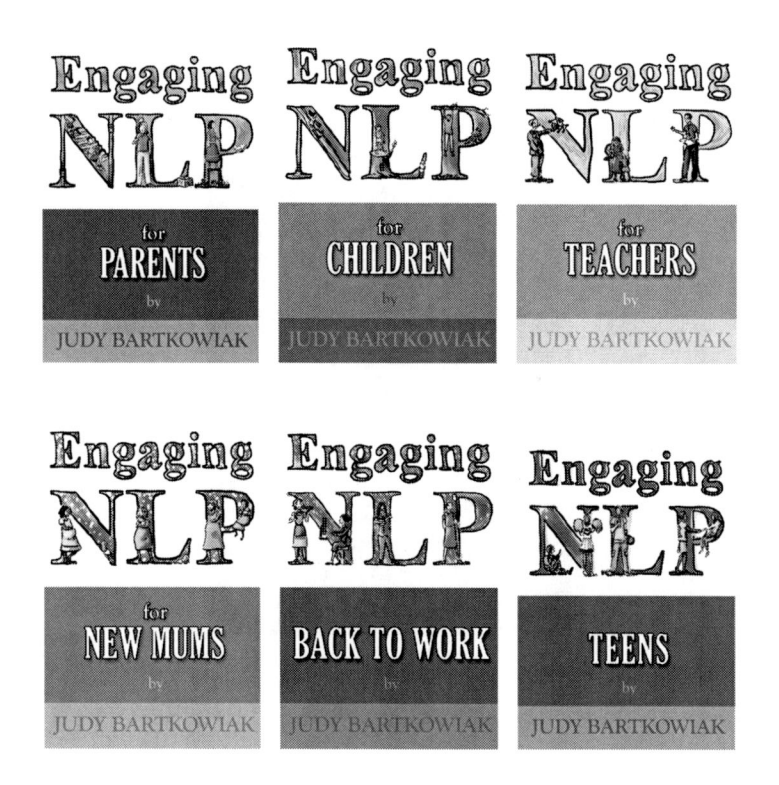

The Engaging NLP series of handbooks bringing simple, practical applications of NLP to everyday life. Parents, Teachers and Children's versions also available in French.

Also From MX Publishing

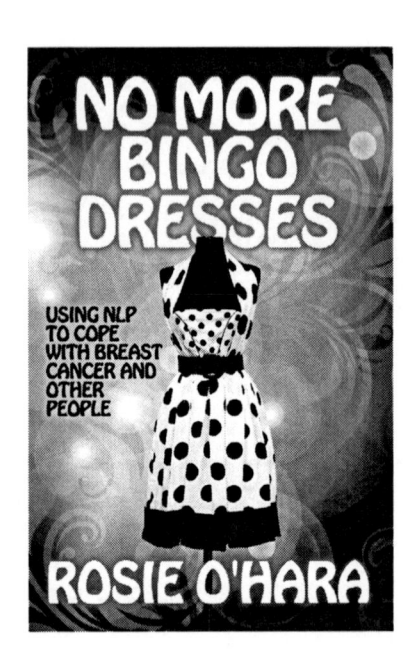

No More Bingo Dresses: Using NLP to cope with breast cancer and other people

Also From MX Publishing

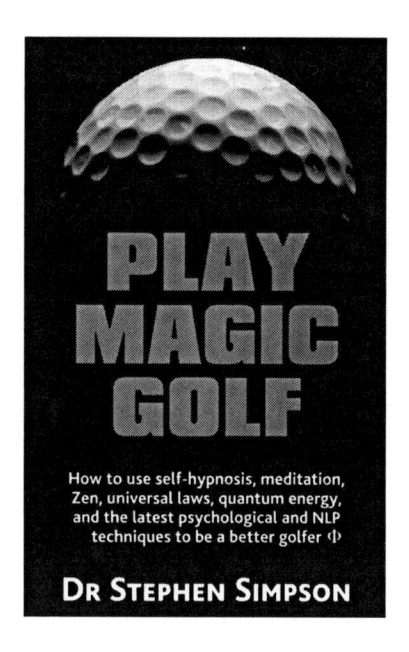

Play Magic Golf: How to use self-hypnosis, meditation, Zen, universal laws, quantum energy, and the latest psychological and NLP techniques to be a better golfer.

Also From MX Publishing

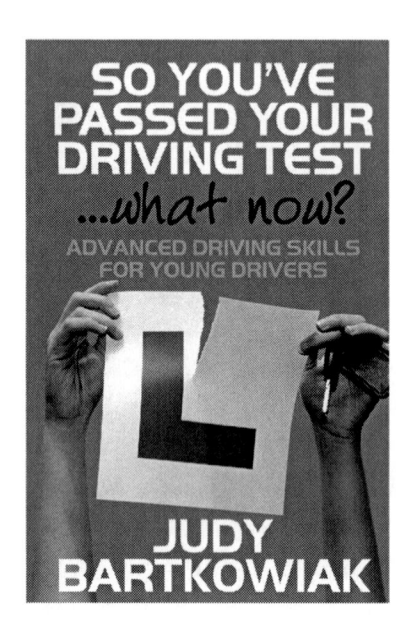

NLP For Young Drivers: Advanced driving skills for young drivers.